HASHIMOTO DIET COOKBOOK

Simple and Delicious Thyroid-Friendly Recipes for Managing Hashimoto's with Food.

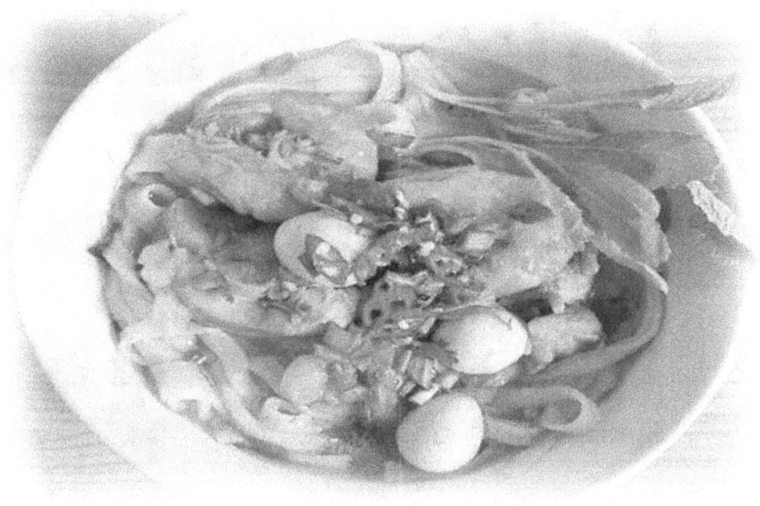

CHRISTIANA WHITE.

GAIN ACCESS TO MORE BOOKS

TABLE OF CONTENTS

INTRODUCTION

In the quiet corners of health difficulties, where murmurs of exhaustion and doubt resound, there is a journey familiar to individuals affected by Hashimoto's. It's a voyage of resilience, adaptation, and the search for a renewed sense of well-being.

Welcome to the world of my Hashimoto Diet Cookbook, a revolutionary guide that has found its way into the lives of many, providing comfort and empowerment to those navigating the maze of Hashimoto's disease.

Each tile represents a person who, armed with the information and sustenance given in these pages, has regained control of their health. These stories are more than just testimonials; they demonstrate the effectiveness of a personalised Hashimoto's diet. As the author, I've walked this journey, faced hardships, and watched successes. This cookbook is more than simply a compilation of recipes; it is a guide on your recovery path.

People who have adopted these recipes have learned that smoothie bowls that awaken the senses can make mornings more energised. They've experienced the satisfaction of delectable lunches that fuel both the body and the spirit, as well as evenings that transform regular meals into self-care routines. Snacks become energising experiences, and desserts become guilt-free celebrations.

The tremendous impact of this cookbook extends beyond the kitchen. It serves as a light of hope for people who have felt the weight of Hashimoto's symptoms, guiding them towards a life free of lethargy, brain fog, and mood swings. Readers have found not only recipes in the pages of this book, but also a comprehensive strategy to controlling their Hashimoto's disease.

Dear reader, as you embark on this journey of nourishment and healing, please know that this cookbook has been thoughtfully designed. It is important to nourish your body, mind, and spirit in addition to what you eat. These recipes contain the keys to achieving energy, resilience, and joy in the face of Hashimoto's.

As you turn the pages, imagine a world in which each meal represents a step towards well-being. Allow this cookbook to be your compass, directing you to a life in which Hashimoto's is not a handicap, but rather a stimulus for a richer, healthier living.

Enter a world where the path to recovery begins in your kitchen. Accept the power of food, the wisdom of this cookbook, and the community of people whose lives have been changed by its transformational enchantment. Welcome to the next phase in your Hashimoto's adventure.

CHAPTER 1

Hashimoto's Disease Overview

As an autoimmune disease, Hashimoto's causes the body's immune system to wrongly target healthy tissues. The thyroid gland, a butterfly-shaped organ in the neck that controls energy levels, metabolism, and a host of other body processes, is the target in this instance.

The most prevalent cause of hypothyroidism, it primarily affects women and affects millions of individuals globally. Prompt diagnosis and treatment are essential to avoid problems.

The symptoms can vary, but they frequently include constipation, cognitive fog, exhaustion, weight gain, hair loss, dry skin, sensitivity to cold, and irregular menstrual periods. Some people, however, might only have minor symptoms or none at all.

Causes: Although the precise reason is yet unknown, gastrointestinal health, genetics, and environmental factors are thought to be involved.

Effects on the Thyroid

Triiodothyronine (T3) and thyroxine (T4) are the two primary hormones produced by the thyroid gland. In other tissues, T4 is transformed into the more active T3. These hormones influence many bodily functions by acting as chemical messengers.

Hashimoto's Attack: In this condition, the thyroid's capacity to generate hormones is diminished because the immune system attacks and damages the thyroid with antibodies. This results in hypothyroidism, a disorder marked by a drop in the levels of T3 and T4 in the blood.

Effects of Hypothyroidism: The body's metabolism slows down when the thyroid produces insufficient hormones, which affects a number of bodily processes. This clarifies the diverse array of symptoms linked to Hashimoto's disease.

The Value of a Dietary Specialisation

Conventional vs. Specialised: Medications to replenish the lost thyroid hormones are part of the traditional treatment for hypothyroidism. Even though they work well, dietary changes can provide further assistance in controlling Hashimoto's and possibly alleviating symptoms.

Dietary Focus: The Hashimoto's diet places special emphasis on certain foods that are meant to promote general health and lower inflammation, both of which are thought to be factors in the autoimmune attack on the thyroid.

Benefits: The diet may assist by introducing particular items and possibly removing others.

- Diminish inflammatory response
- Enhance digestive health, as this might affect immunity
- Consume more nutrients to help the thyroid operate.
- Boost vitality and general well-being

Recall that although the special diet shows promise, it cannot take the place of medication. For best outcomes, it is imperative to collaborate with a healthcare provider to create a customised strategy that incorporates nutritional and medical management.

CHAPTER 2

The Hashimoto's Diet's Basics

The Hashimoto's diet is a set of dietary guidelines designed to optimize nutritional intake, reduce inflammation, and support gut health in order to improve thyroid function and general well-being. It is not a single, strict plan. It highlights:

• **Complete, unprocessed foods**: Complex carbs, lean proteins, healthy fats, and fruits and vegetables are good sources of fibre and vital nutrients.

• **Anti-inflammatory foods**: These include leafy greens, berries, and fatty fish. They also contain antioxidants and other substances that help reduce inflammation.

• **Foods that heal the gut**: Prebiotics and fermented foods support a balanced gut microbiota, which boosts immunity.

• **Nutrient-dense foods**: Paying attention to vitamins, minerals, and vital fatty acids promotes thyroid health and general well-being.

Foods to Include or Avoid:

Add:

- Colourful fruits and vegetables, such as cruciferous vegetables, leafy greens, and berries, are high in fibre and antioxidants.

- Lean Proteins: Chicken, fish (tuna, salmon), beans, lentils, eggs (if permitted), and poultry
- Nuts, seeds, avocados, olive oil, and flaxseed oil are good sources of fat.
- Complex Carbohydrates: Sweet potatoes, lentils, and whole grains (quinoa, brown rice).
- Fermented foods: sauerkraut, kimchi, kefir, and yogurt
- Herbs and Spices: cinnamon, ginger, garlic, and turmeric

Don't:

- Gluten: If you are sensitive to gluten, think about choosing gluten-free products since these may help reduce inflammation in certain people.
- Dairy: Like gluten, dairy can make some people feel irritated. Try substitutes like yogurt made from goat milk or plant-based milks.
- Refined carbohydrates and added sugars: They increase blood sugar swings and inflammation. Cut back on processed foods, white bread, sweetened beverages, and pastries.
- Nightshades: For certain people, foods including potatoes, tomatoes, peppers, and eggplant might exacerbate inflammation. Think about eliminating if you have problems.

- Soy: May hinder the absorption of thyroid hormones; moderation or avoidance may be advised.
- Food Sensitivities: Remove triggers and observe how each person responds to different foods.

Relationship between Thyroid Health and Nutrition

Although studies are still being conducted, new data points to a connection between nutrition and thyroid function in Hashimoto's:

• **Inflammation:** Food can have an effect on the long-term inflammation linked to Hashimoto's disease. Foods that are anti-inflammatory may aid in reducing inflammation and perhaps enhance thyroid function.

• **Gut Health:** Autoimmune diseases are associated with a gut microbiome that is important for the immune system. Foods that heal the gut may help maintain a balanced microbiota and boost immunity.

• **Nutrient Deficiencies**: Iron, zinc, and iodine deficiencies, among others, can have an impact on thyroid function. Nutrient-rich foods are the focus of the Hashimoto's diet in order to guarantee optimal intake.

Crucial Information:

- Reactions to the Hashimoto's diet can differ from person to person. Observe your body and make any necessary adjustments.
- The diet should be used in conjunction with medication and medical advice as it is not a cure-all.
- For individualized advice, speak with a qualified dietitian or other medical practitioner.

The Hashimoto's diet can be an effective tool for treating your condition and enhancing general well-being if you incorporate these ideas and modify it to suit your unique circumstances. Keep in mind that this is a journey, not a destination, and the secret is to figure out what works best for you!

CHAPTER 3

Breakfast

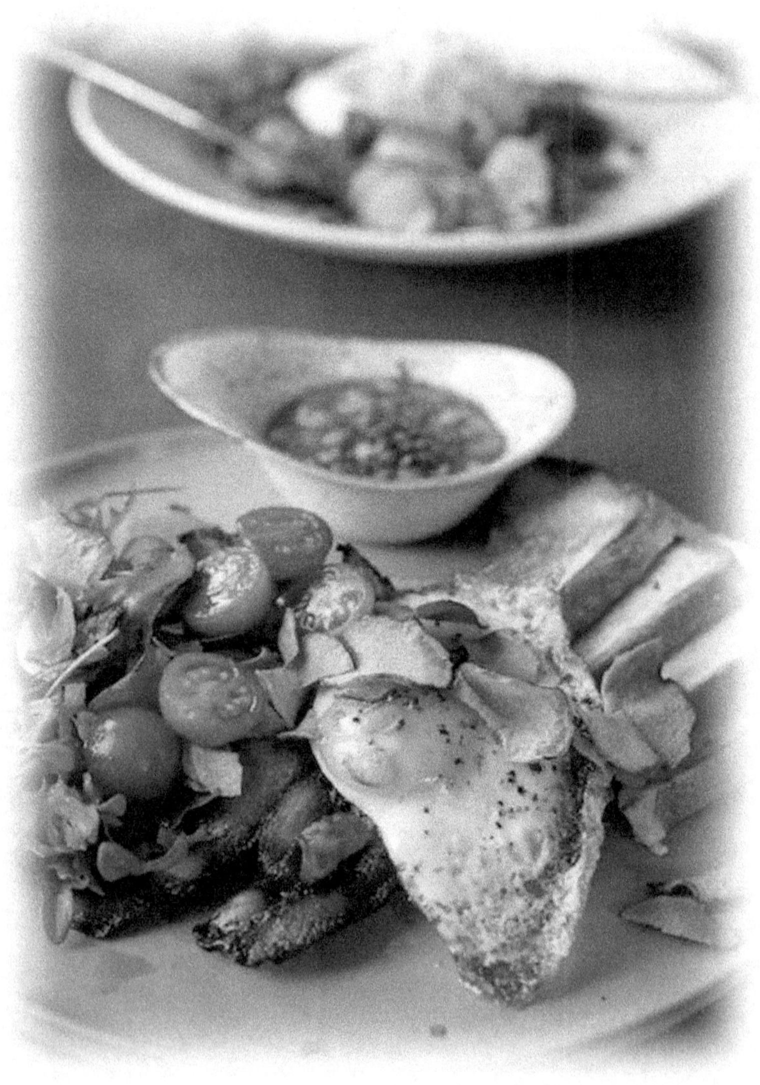

Antioxidant Smoothie Bowl.

- **Serves: 1**
- **Prep time is 10 minutes.**

Ingredients:

- 1 cup frozen mixed berries.
- 1/2 cup unsweetened almond milk.
- One-quarter cup plain coconut yogurt
- One spoonful of chia seeds.
- One-quarter teaspoon of vanilla extract
- Optional toppings include fresh berries, sliced almonds, shredded coconut, hemp seeds, and more.

Instructions

- In a blender, mix together the frozen berries, almond milk, coconut yogurt, chia seeds, and vanilla extract. Blend until smooth and creamy.
- Pour the smoothie into a bowl and add any preferred toppings.
- Enjoy your antioxidant smoothie bowl!

Nutritional values per serving:

- Calories: 320.
- Protein: 9 grams.
- Fibre: 15 grams.

Scrambled Eggs with Avocado and Smoked Salmon.

- **Servings: Two.**
- **Prepare time: 15 minutes.**

Ingredients

- 4 eggs
- Two teaspoons of water.
- Salt and pepper to taste.
- One tablespoon of coconut oil.
- One ripe avocado, peeled and sliced
- 4 oz. smoked salmon, sliced
- Optional garnishes include fresh dill, lemon wedges, and so forth.

Instructions

- In a small bowl, mix together the eggs, water, salt, and pepper.
- Melt the coconut oil in a large skillet over medium-high heat, then swirl to coat.
- Pour the egg mixture into the pan and heat, stirring regularly, for about 10 minutes, or until the eggs set.
- Divide the scrambled eggs amongst two plates, then top with avocado and smoked salmon pieces.
- Optional garnishes include fresh dill and lemon wedges.

- Top your scrambled eggs with avocado and smoked salmon.

Nutritional values per serving:

- Calories: 470.

- Protein: 29 grams

- Healthy fats: 36 grams

Chia Pudding with Coconut Milk and Mango

- **Servings: two.**

- **Prep time: 5 minutes, including overnight chilling.**

Ingredients

- 1/4 cup chia seeds.

- One cup full-fat coconut milk.

- 2 tablespoons pure maple syrup.

- 1/2 teaspoon vanilla extract.

- 1/4 teaspoon ground cardamom.

- One ripe mango, peeled and diced

- Optional toppings include toasted coconut flakes, chopped pistachios, and more.

Instructions

- In a medium mixing bowl, blend the chia seeds, coconut milk, maple syrup, vanilla essence, and cardamom until thoroughly incorporated.

- Cover the bowl and chill overnight, or at least 4 hours, until the chia seeds have absorbed the liquid and created a pudding-like texture.
- In the morning, stir the chia pudding and divide it into two dishes or jars.
- Garnish with diced mango and desired toppings.
- Enjoy chia pudding with coconut milk and mango!

Nutritional values per serving:

- Calories: 410.
- Protein: 7 grams.
- Fibre: 13 grams.

Oatmeal with Berries and Nuts

- **Servings: two.**
- **Prepare time: 15 minutes.**

Ingredients

- 1 cup gluten-free rolled oats.
- Two glasses of water.
- One pinch of salt.
- 1/4 teaspoon ground cinnamon.
- 2 tablespoons pure maple syrup.
- 1/2 cup fresh or frozen mixed berries.
- 1/4 cup chopped walnuts or pecans.

- Optional toppings include almond butter, coconut yogurt, hemp seeds, and more.

Instructions

- Heat the oats, water, salt, and cinnamon in a small saucepan over medium-high heat until boiling. Reduce the heat to a simmer, stirring occasionally, for about 10 minutes, or until the oats are soft and creamy.
- Add the maple syrup and remove from heat.
- Divide the oats into two portions and top with berries and nuts.
- Top your oats with fruit and nuts!

Nutritional values per serving:

- Total calories: 360.
- Protein: 9 grams.
- Fibre: 8 grams.

Sweet Potato Hash and Eggs

- **Servings: four.**
- **Prepare time: 30 minutes.**

Ingredients

- Two medium sweet potatoes, peeled and diced
- Two teaspoons of coconut oil.
- Salt and pepper to taste.
- 1/4 teaspoon smoked paprika.

- One-quarter teaspoon of garlic powder
- 4 eggs
- Optional garnishes include fresh parsley, spicy sauce, and so forth.

Instructions

- Preheat the oven to 200°C (180°C fan-forced) and prepare a baking sheet with parchment paper.
- Toss the sweet potatoes in a large bowl with 1 tablespoon coconut oil, salt, pepper, smoky paprika, and garlic powder until thoroughly coated.
- Place the sweet potatoes in an even layer on the prepared baking sheet and bake for 20 minutes, flipping halfway through, until soft and golden.
- Heat the remaining 1 tablespoon coconut oil in a large oven-safe skillet over medium-high heat, then crack in the eggs, allowing some space between them. Season with salt and pepper and cook for 5 minutes, or until the whites are firm but the yolks are still runny.
- Place the skillet in the oven for a further 5 minutes, or until the eggs are cooked to your preference.
- If wanted, serve the eggs over the sweet potato hash and sprinkle with fresh parsley and spicy sauce.
- Enjoy sweet potato hash with eggs!

Nutritional values per serving:

- Calories: 280.

- Protein: 11 grams.

- Vitamin A (260% DV)

Quinoa Porridge with Cinnamon and Apples.

- **Servings: four.**

- **Prep time is 25 minutes.**

Ingredients

- 1 cup quinoa, washed and drained.

- Two glasses of water.

- One cup of unsweetened almond milk.

- 2 tablespoons pure maple syrup.

- One teaspoon of ground cinnamon.

- 1/4 teaspoon ground nutmeg.

- Two apples, cored and diced

- Optional toppings include chopped almonds, raisins, and coconut flakes.

Instructions

- Heat the quinoa and water in a medium saucepan over high heat until boiling. Reduce the heat to a simmer and cover for about 15 minutes, or until the quinoa is fluffy and the water has been absorbed.

- Add the almond milk, maple syrup, cinnamon, and nutmeg, and bring to a boil again.
- Reduce the heat to a simmer, stirring occasionally, until the porridge is thick and creamy, about 10 minutes.
- Cook the apples in a small skillet over medium-high heat, turning constantly, until softened and caramelized, about 15 minutes.
- Divide the quinoa porridge among four bowls, then top with the cooked apples and any desired toppings.
- Top your quinoa porridge with cinnamon and apples.

Nutritional values per serving:

- Calories: 310.
- Protein: 9 grams.
- Iron: 15% DV.

Gluten-Free Pancakes with Banana and Nut Butter

- **Servings: two.**
- **Prep time is 20 minutes.**

Ingredients

- One ripe banana, mashed
- 2 eggs
- One-quarter cup almond flour

- One-quarter teaspoon of baking powder

- One pinch of salt.

- One tablespoon of coconut oil.

- 2 tablespoons of your preferred nut butter (almond, peanut, or cashew)

- Optional toppings include sliced banana, pure maple syrup, chocolate chips, and more.

Instructions

- In a larger bowl, combine the banana, eggs, almond flour, baking powder, and salt.

- Melt the coconut oil in a large non-stick skillet over medium-low heat, then drop about 1/4 cup batter onto each pancake.

- Cook for 3 minutes, or until bubbles appear on the surface, then flipping and cooking for another 2 minutes, or until golden and cooked through.

- Repeat with the remaining batter, using extra coconut oil as needed.

- Drizzle the nut butter over the pancakes and top with any desired toppings.

- Enjoy your gluten-free pancakes with bananas and nut butter!

Nutritional values per serving:

- Calories:420

- Protein: 16 grams

- Calcium (10% DV)

Green Smoothie with Kale, Apple, And Ginger.

- **Servings: two.**
- **Prep time is 10 minutes.**

Ingredients

- Two cups of chopped kale.
- One large apple, cored and cut
- 1/2-inch fresh ginger, peeled and minced.
- Two glasses of water.
- Two teaspoons of lemon juice.
- Two teaspoons of honey.
- Optional ingredients: ice cubes, protein powder, flax seeds, etc.

Instructions

- In a blender, mix the kale, apple, ginger, water, lemon juice, and honey. Blend until smooth and frothy.
- Add any optional ingredients and blend again until thoroughly combined.
- Pour the smoothie into two glasses and enjoy your green kale, apple, and ginger smoothie!

Nutritional values per serving:

- Calories: 140.

- Protein: 3 grams.

- Vitamin K: 600% DV.

Baked Tofu Scramble with Vegetables.

- **Servings: four.**

- **Prep time is 40 minutes.**

Ingredients

- Drain and crumble one block (14 ounces) of firm tofu.

- Two tablespoons of nutritional yeast.

- One teaspoon of turmeric.

- A half teaspoon of salt.

- 1/4 teaspoon black pepper.

- Two teaspoons of coconut oil.

- 1 onion, chopped

- 2 garlic cloves, minced

- Two cups of chopped kale.

- One cup cherry tomato, halved

- Optional garnishes include fresh parsley, avocado slices, and so on.

Instructions

- Preheat the oven to 180°C (160°C fan-forced) and gently butter a 9x13-inch baking pan.
- In a large bowl, combine the tofu, nutritional yeast, turmeric, salt, and pepper.
- Spread the tofu mixture evenly in the prepared baking dish, then bake for 25 minutes, or until golden and firm.
- Heat the coconut oil in a large skillet over medium-high heat, then sauté the onion and garlic until tender, about 15 minutes.
- Cook, stirring periodically, until the kale wilts and the tomatoes soften, about 10 minutes.
- Serve the tofu scramble with the vegetable mixture, topped with fresh parsley and avocado slices if desired.
- Enjoy your baked tofu scramble with vegetables.

Nutritional values per serving:

- Calories: 260
- Protein: 18 grams
- Vitamin C: 70% of the daily value

Coconut Yogurt Parfait with Granola and Berries

- **Servings: two.**
- **Prep time is 10 minutes.**

Ingredients

- One cup plain coconut yogurt.
- 2 tablespoons pure maple syrup.
- 1/2 teaspoon vanilla extract.
- 1/4 teaspoon ground cinnamon.
- One cup of gluten-free granola.
- 1 cup fresh or frozen mixed berries.
- Optional toppings include shredded coconut, chopped almonds, and more.

Instructions

- In a small bowl, whisk together the coconut yogurt, maple syrup, vanilla essence, and cinnamon until thoroughly incorporated.
- Layer the yogurt, granola, and berries in two glasses or jars, alternating until all of the ingredients are utilized.
- Add your favourite toppings and enjoy your coconut yogurt parfait with granola and berries!

Nutritional values per serving:

- Calories: 440
- Protein: 8 grams.
- Calcium: 15% DV.

CHAPTER 4

<u>Lunch</u>

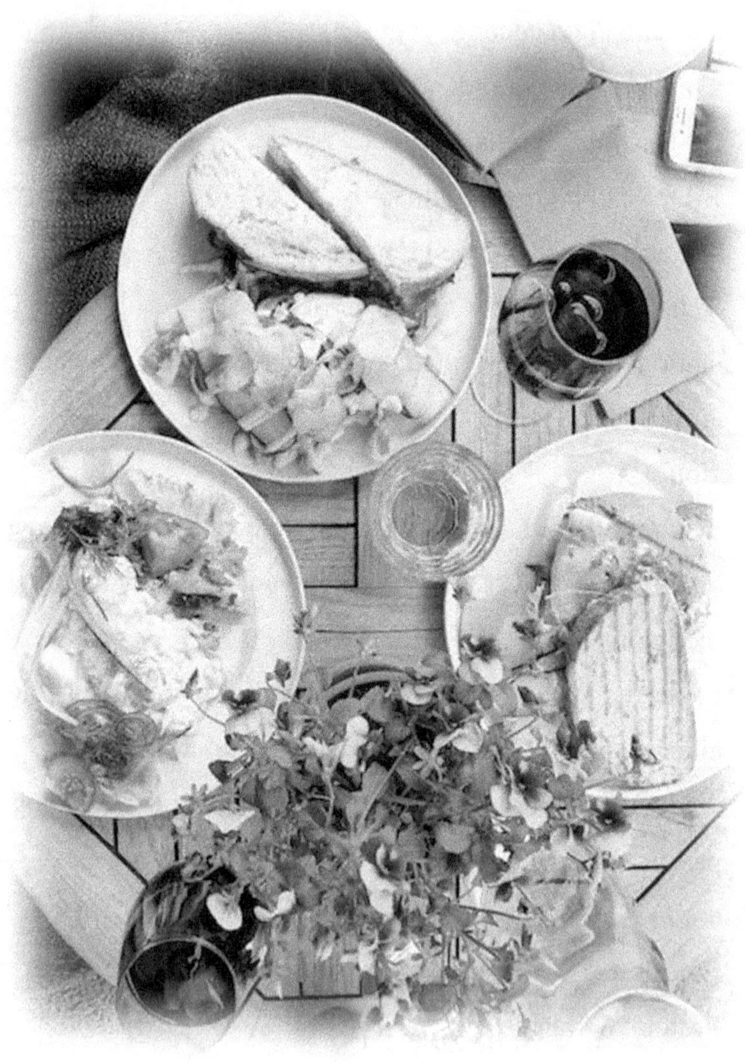

Salmon Salad with Quinoa and Roasted Vegetables.

- **Servings: four.**
- **Prep time is 40 minutes.**

Ingredients

- 1 cup quinoa, washed and drained.
- Two glasses of water.
- Salt and pepper to taste.
- Four (4-ounce) salmon fillets.
- Two teaspoons of olive oil.
- Two teaspoons of dried rosemary.
- 4 cups of chopped mixed veggies, including broccoli, cauliflower, carrots, and zucchini.
- 1/4 cup chopped fresh parsley.
- Two teaspoons of lemon juice.
- Optional dressings include simple coconut yogurt, Dijon mustard, honey, and so forth.

Instructions

- Preheat the oven to 200°C (180°C fan-forced) and prepare two baking sheets with parchment paper.
- Heat the quinoa, water, and a pinch of salt in a small skillet over high heat until boiling.

- Reduce the heat to a simmer and cover for about 15 minutes, or until the quinoa is fluffy and the water has been absorbed. Fluff with a fork, then set aside.
- In a small bowl, combine the olive oil, rosemary, salt, and pepper. Brush half of the oil mixture onto the salmon fillets and place on one of the prepared baking pans.
- Bake for 15 minutes, or until the salmon is well cooked and readily flaked with a fork.
- Toss the vegetables with the remaining oil mixture and spread on the other baking sheet. Bake for 20 minutes, or until the veggies have softened and roasted.
- In a large bowl, combine the quinoa, parsley, and lemon juice. Season with salt and pepper as needed.
- Serve the salmon fillets with quinoa and roasted veggies. Drizzle with your preferred dressing, if using.
- Pair your salmon salad with quinoa and roasted vegetables.

Nutritional values per serving:
- Calories: 480.
- Protein: 35 grams
- Omega-3 fatty acids: 2 grams

Lentil Soup with Whole Wheat Bread

- **Servings: six.**
- **Prep time is 50 minutes.**

Ingredients

- Two teaspoons of coconut oil.
- 1 onion, chopped
- Two carrots, peeled and chopped
- Two celery stalks, diced
- 4 garlic cloves, minced
- One teaspoon of cumin.
- 1/2 teaspoon turmeric.
- 1/4 teaspoon smoked paprika.
- Salt and pepper to taste.
- Six cups of veggie broth.
- Rinse and drain 2 cups of brown lentils.
- Two bay leaves.
- Two teaspoons of apple cider vinegar.
- Optional garnishes include fresh parsley, coconut yogurt, and so forth.
- Six pieces of whole wheat bread.

Instructions

- Heat the coconut oil in a big pot over medium-high heat. Sauté the onion, carrots, celery, and garlic for around 15 minutes.

- Add the cumin, turmeric, smoked paprika, salt, and pepper and simmer for another minute, until aromatic.
- Bring the vegetable broth, lentils, and bay leaves to a boil. Reduce the heat and simmer, slightly covered, for about 25 minutes, or until the lentils are cooked.
- Discard the bay leaves and add the apple cider vinegar. If needed, season with additional salt and pepper.
- Ladle the soup into dishes and top with fresh parsley and coconut yogurt, if desired.
- Enjoy your lentil soup with whole wheat toast!

Nutritional values per serving:

- Total calories: 360.
- Protein: 18 grams
- Fibre: 16 grams.

Chicken Lettuce Wraps with Avocado and Mango Salsa.

- **Servings: four.**
- **Prepare time: 30 minutes.**

Ingredients

- One ripe avocado, peeled and diced
- One ripe mango, peeled and diced
- 1/4 cup chopped fresh cilantro.

- Two teaspoons of lime juice.

- Salt and pepper to taste.

- One tablespoon of coconut oil.

- Cut 1 pound of boneless, skinless chicken breasts into bite-sized pieces.

- One teaspoon of chili powder.

- 1/2 teaspoon cumin.

- One-quarter teaspoon of garlic powder

- 12 large lettuce leaves (romaine or butter lettuce)

- Optional toppings include shredded cabbage, sliced radishes, and more.

Instructions

- In a medium bowl, combine the avocado, mango, cilantro, and lime juice. Season with salt and pepper to taste. Refrigerate until ready to serve.

- Heat the coconut oil in a large skillet over medium-high heat, then cook the chicken pieces for about 15 minutes, tossing regularly, until browned and well cooked.

- Toss the chicken with the chili powder, cumin, garlic powder, salt, and pepper until coated.

- To assemble the wraps, spread some chicken and avocado-mango salsa on each lettuce leaf. Add your favourite toppings and enjoy your chicken lettuce wraps with avocado and mango salsa!

Nutritional values per serving:

- Calories: 320.

- Protein: 28 grams

- Vitamin C: 60% DV.

Black Bean Burgers with Gluten-Free Buns

- **Servings: four.**

- **Prepare time: 30 minutes.**

Ingredients

- One (15-ounce) can of black beans, drained and rinsed

- 1/4 cup gluten-free oats.

- 2 teaspoons of chopped fresh cilantro.

- One teaspoon of cumin.

- One-half teaspoon of garlic powder

- Salt and pepper to taste.

- One tablespoon of coconut oil.

- 4 gluten-free, toasted buns

- Optional toppings include lettuce, tomato, onion, avocado, salsa, and more.

Instructions

- In a food processor, add the black beans, oats, cilantro, cumin, garlic powder, salt, and pepper. Process until well incorporated but still slightly chunky.

- Shape the mixture into four patties and chill for 15 minutes to harden.

- Heat the coconut oil in a big skillet over medium-high heat. Cook the patties for about 4 minutes on each side, or until brown and crisp.

- To assemble the burgers, lay a patty on each bun and top with your favourite toppings.

- Enjoy your black bean burgers on gluten-free buns!

Nutritional values per serving:

- Calories: 300.

- Protein: 12 grams.

- Fibre: 10 grams.

Turkey and Vegetable Stir-Fry with Brown Rice.

- **Servings: four.**

- **Prepare time: 30 minutes.**

Ingredients

- One cup brown rice.

- Two glasses of water.

- Salt to taste.

- One tablespoon of coconut oil.

- One pound of ground turkey.

- 2 tablespoons of minced ginger.

- 2 garlic cloves, minced

- 1/4 teaspoon red pepper flakes.

- 2 cups broccoli florets.

- One red bell pepper, sliced

- 1/4 cup coconut aminos.

- Two teaspoons of apple cider vinegar.

- One spoonful of honey.

- One tablespoon of sesame seeds.

- Optional garnishes include sliced green onions and minced cilantro.

Instructions

- Heat the rice, water, and a pinch of salt in a small skillet over high heat until boiling. Reduce the heat to a simmer and cover for about 20 minutes, or until the rice is cooked and the water has been absorbed. Fluff with a fork, then set aside.

- Heat the coconut oil in a big skillet over medium-high heat. Cook the turkey, breaking it up with a spatula, until it is browned and cooked through, about 15 minutes.

- Drain the excess grease and place the turkey on a plate.

- In the same skillet, sauté the ginger, garlic, and red pepper flakes until fragrant, about 1 minute.

- Bring the broccoli, bell pepper, coconut aminos, vinegar, and honey to a boil.

- Reduce the heat to a simmer, stirring periodically, for about 10 minutes, or until the veggies are crisp tender.

- Return the turkey to the skillet and stir to mix. Sprinkle with sesame seeds and, if preferred, add green onions and cilantro.
- Serve the turkey and veggie stir-fry with brown rice and enjoy!

Nutritional values per serving:

• **Calories:420**

• **Protein: 30 grams.**

• **Fibre: 5 grams.**

Chickpea Salad Sandwich on Whole Wheat Bread.

- **Servings: four.**
- **Prepare time: 15 minutes.**

Ingredients

- 1 (15-ounce) can drained and washed chickpeas.
- One-quarter cup plain coconut yogurt
- 2 teaspoons of Dijon mustard.
- One-quarter teaspoon of salt
- 1/4 teaspoon black pepper.
- 2 teaspoons of chopped fresh dill.
- Two celery stalks, diced
- 1/4 cup chopped walnuts.

- Eight pieces of whole wheat bread.
- Optional toppings include lettuce, tomato, and cucumber.

Instructions

- In a large mixing bowl, mash the chickpeas with a fork or a potato masher until somewhat lumpy.
- Combine the coconut yogurt, mustard, salt, pepper, dill, celery, and walnuts and mix thoroughly.
- To make the sandwiches, spread chickpea salad over four slices of bread. Add your favourite toppings, then top with another slice of bread.
- Cut the sandwiches in half and devour your chickpea salad sandwich on whole wheat bread!

Nutritional values per serving:

- Calories: 380.
- Protein: 16 grams
- Iron (20% DV)

Tuna Salad with Mixed Greens and Avocado.

- **Servings: four.**
- **Prepare time: 15 minutes.**

Ingredients

- Two 5-ounce cans of tuna, drained and flaked.
- One-quarter cup plain coconut yogurt
- Two teaspoons of lemon juice.

- One-quarter teaspoon of salt
- 1/4 teaspoon black pepper.
- 2 teaspoons of freshly chopped parsley.
- Four cups of mixed greens, including spinach, kale, and arugula.
- One ripe avocado, peeled and sliced
- Optional dressings include olive oil, apple cider vinegar, and honey.

Instructions

- In a medium mixing bowl, combine the tuna, coconut yogurt, lemon juice, salt, pepper, and parsley until well blended.
- Divide the mixed greens across four dishes, then top with the tuna mixture and avocado slices.
- Drizzle with your preferred dressing, if using.
- Pair your tuna salad with mixed greens and avocado.

Nutritional values per serving:

- Calories: 240
- Protein: 22 grams
- Healthy fats: 12 grams

Vegetarian Chili with Brown Rice and Cornbread.

- **Servings: six.**
- **Prep time is 50 minutes.**

Ingredients

- One tablespoon of coconut oil.
- 1 onion, chopped
- One red bell pepper, chopped
- 2 garlic cloves, minced
- Two teaspoons of chili powder.
- One teaspoon of cumin.
- 1/2 teaspoons of smoked paprika.
- Salt and pepper to taste.
- 1 can (28 ounces) of diced tomatoes
- One (15-ounce) can of black beans, drained and rinsed
- One (15-ounce) can of kidney beans, drained and rinsed
- One cup of veggie broth.
- Two tablespoons of tomato paste.
- One tablespoon of apple cider vinegar.
- Optional garnishes include shredded cheese, sour cream, and green onions.
- Three cups cooked brown rice.
- One (8.5-ounce) package of gluten-free cornbread mix.
- 1 egg
- One-third cup coconut oil

- 2/3 cup unsweetened almond milk.

Instructions

- Preheat the oven to 180°C (160°C fan-forced) and lightly butter an 8x8-inch baking pan.
- Heat the coconut oil in a large saucepan over medium-high heat. Sauté the onion, bell pepper, garlic, chili powder, cumin, smoky paprika, salt, and pepper until tender, about 15 minutes.
- Add the tomatoes, black beans, kidney beans, broth, tomato paste, and vinegar, and bring to a boil.
- Reduce the heat and let the chili to simmer, uncovered, for about 20 minutes, or until thick and flavourful.
- In a large mixing bowl, combine the cornbread mix, egg, coconut oil, and almond milk until thoroughly blended.
- Place the mixture in the prepared baking sheet and bake for 20 minutes, or until brown and a toothpick inserted in the centre comes out clean.
- Serve the chili over rice and cornbread. Garnish with cheese, sour cream, and green onions as desired.
- Pair your vegetarian chili with brown rice and cornbread.

Nutritional values per serving:

- Calories: 560
- Protein: 16 grams
- Fibre: 14 grams.

Quinoa Salad with Roasted Sweet Potatoes and Black Beans.

- **Servings: four.**
- **Prep time is 40 minutes.**

Ingredients

- One large sweet potato, peeled and diced
- Two teaspoons of olive oil.
- Salt and pepper to taste.
- 1 cup quinoa, washed and drained.
- Two glasses of water.
- One (15-ounce) can of black beans, drained and rinsed
- 1/4 cup chopped fresh cilantro.
- Two teaspoons of lime juice.
- One teaspoon of cumin.
- One-quarter teaspoon of garlic powder
- Optional toppings include avocado, feta cheese, pumpkin seeds, and more.

Instructions

- Preheat the oven to 200°C (180°C fan-forced) and prepare a baking sheet with parchment paper.
- Toss the sweet potato in a large mixing dish with 1 tablespoon olive oil, salt, and pepper until thoroughly coated.

- Place the sweet potatoes in an even layer on the prepared baking sheet and bake for 20 minutes, flipping halfway through, until soft and golden.
- Heat the quinoa, water, and a pinch of salt in a small skillet over high heat until boiling. Reduce the heat to a simmer and cover for about 15 minutes, or until the quinoa is fluffy and the water has been absorbed. Fluff with a fork, then set aside.

- In a large bowl, combine the remaining 1 tablespoon olive oil, cilantro, lime juice, cumin, garlic powder, salt, and pepper.
- Toss together the quinoa, black beans, and roasted sweet potatoes.
- Serve the quinoa salad with your preferred toppings and enjoy!

Nutritional values per serving:
- Calories:420
- Protein: 15 grams.
- Iron: 25% DV.

Leftover Turkey and Vegetable Soup with Whole-Grain Crackers.

- **Servings: six.**
- **Prepare time: 30 minutes.**

Ingredients

- Two teaspoons of coconut oil.
- 1 onion, chopped
- Two carrots, peeled and sliced
- Two celery stalks, diced
- 4 garlic cloves, minced
- Salt and pepper to taste.
- Six cups of turkey or chicken broth.
- Two cups of shredded leftover turkey.
- 2 cups of mixed veggies, including green beans, corn, and peas.
- 2 teaspoons of freshly chopped parsley.
- Optional garnishes include shredded cheese, sour cream, and other ingredients.
- 24 whole grain crackers.

Instructions

- Heat the coconut oil in a big pot over medium-high heat. Sauté the onion, carrots, celery, and garlic for around 15 minutes. Season with salt and pepper to taste.

- Bring the soup to a boil by adding the stock, turkey, and mixed vegetables.
- Reduce the heat to a simmer, uncovered, for about 15 minutes, or until the vegetables are soft.
- Stir in the parsley and adjust seasoning as needed.
- Ladle the soup into bowls and top with cheese and sour cream, if preferred.
- Enjoy leftover turkey and vegetable soup with whole-grain crackers!

Nutritional values per serving:

- Calories: 340.
- Protein: 24 grams
- Fibre: 6 grams.

CHAPTER 5

Dinner

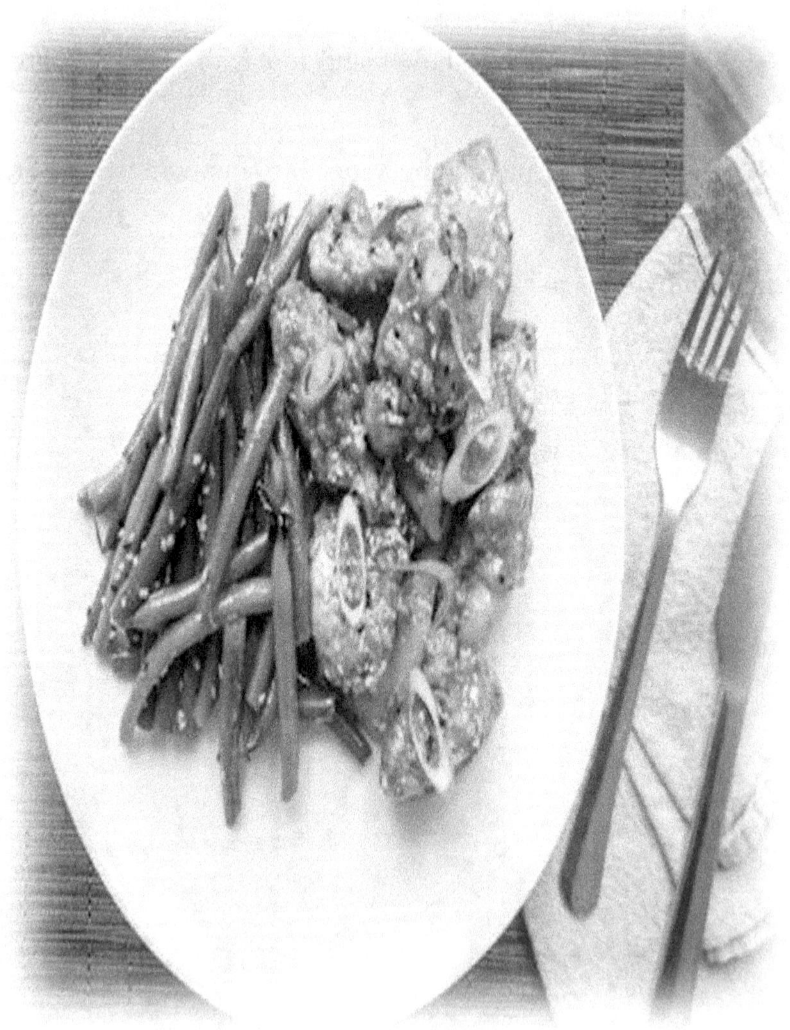

Baked Salmon with Roasted Brussels Sprouts And Quinoa.

- **Servings: four.**
- **Prep time is 40 minutes.**

Ingredients

- Four (4-ounce) salmon fillets.
- Two teaspoons of olive oil.
- Salt and pepper to taste.
- Two teaspoons dried thyme.
- 4 cups trimmed and halved Brussels sprouts.
- 1 cup quinoa, washed and drained.
- Two glasses of water.
- 1/4 cup chopped fresh parsley.
- Two teaspoons of lemon juice.

Instructions

- Preheat the oven to 200°C (180°C fan-forced) and prepare a baking sheet with parchment paper.
- In a small bowl, combine 1 tablespoon olive oil, salt, pepper, and thyme. Brush the salmon fillets with the oil mixture and arrange them on one end of the prepared baking sheet. Bake for 15 minutes, or until the salmon is well cooked and readily flaked with a fork.

- Toss the Brussels sprouts in a large basin with the remaining 1 tablespoon olive oil, salt, and pepper until evenly coated. Spread them out on the other end of the prepared baking sheet and roast for 20 minutes, or until soft.
- Heat the quinoa, water, and a pinch of salt in a small skillet over high heat until boiling.
- Reduce the heat to a simmer and cover for about 15 minutes, or until the quinoa is fluffy and the water has been absorbed.
- Fluff with a fork, then whisk in the parsley and lemon juice. Season with salt and pepper as needed.
- Enjoy your baked salmon with quinoa and roasted Brussels sprouts!

Nutritional values per serving:

- Calories: 480.
- Protein: 35 grams
- Omega-3 fatty acids: 2 grams

Chicken Curry with Coconut Milk and Vegetables

- **Servings: four.**
- **Prepare time: 30 minutes.**

Ingredients

- One tablespoon of coconut oil.
- 1 onion, chopped
- 2 garlic cloves, minced

- 1 tablespoon of minced ginger.

- Two teaspoons of curry powder.

- One teaspoon of turmeric.

- A half teaspoon of salt.

- 1/4 teaspoon black pepper.

- One (13.5-ounce) can of full-fat coconut milk.

- One-quarter cup vegetable broth

- Cut 1 pound of boneless, skinless chicken breasts into bite-sized pieces.

- 2 cups of mixed veggies, such as cauliflower, carrots, and peas

- 2 teaspoons of chopped fresh cilantro.

- Optional garnish: lime wedges, extra cilantro, etc.

- 4 cups of cooked brown rice

Instructions

- In a large skillet over medium-high heat, heat the coconut oil and sauté the onion, garlic, ginger, curry powder, turmeric, salt, and pepper until tender and aromatic, about 15 minutes.

- Stir in the coconut milk and broth and bring the mixture to a boil. Reduce the heat and simmer, stirring periodically, until slightly thickened, about 10 minutes.

- Add the chicken and veggies and simmer, stirring periodically, until the chicken is cooked through and the vegetables are soft, about 15 minutes.

- Stir in the cilantro and adjust the seasoning, if needed.
- Serve the chicken curry over the rice and garnish with lime wedges and extra cilantro, if preferred.
- Enjoy your chicken curry with coconut milk and vegetables!

Nutritional values per serving:

- Calories: 520
- Protein: 32 g
- Fibre: 6 grams.

One-Pan Lemon Herb Shrimp with Roasted Asparagus

- **Servings: four.**
- **Prep time is 25 minutes.**

Ingredients

- One pound of big shrimp, peeled and deveined
- Two teaspoons of olive oil.
- Two teaspoons of dried oregano.
- One teaspoon dried basil.
- Salt and pepper to taste.
- One lemon, cut
- One bunch of asparagus, trimmed and divided into thirds
- 2 teaspoons of freshly chopped parsley.

- Optional garnishes include lemon wedges, more parsley, and so forth.

Instructions

- Preheat the oven to 200°C (180°C fan-forced) and prepare a baking sheet with parchment paper.
- Toss the shrimp in a large bowl with 1 tablespoon olive oil, oregano, basil, salt, and pepper until thoroughly coated.
- Place the shrimp and lemon slices in a single layer on one end of the prepared baking sheet.
- Toss the asparagus in the same bowl with the remaining 1 tablespoon olive oil, salt, and pepper until evenly coated. Arrange the asparagus at the other end of the prepared baking sheet.
- Bake for 15 minutes, or until the shrimp become pink and the asparagus is soft.
- Garnish with lemon wedges and more parsley, if desired.
- Enjoy your one-pan lemon herb shrimp and roasted asparagus!

Nutritional values per serving:

- Calories: 260
- Protein: 25 grams
- Vitamin A: 15% DV.

Turkey Meatloaf with Sweet Potato Mash and Green Beans.

- **Servings: four.**
- **Prep time is 60 minutes.**

Ingredients

- One pound of ground turkey.
- A quarter cup of gluten-free breadcrumbs
- 1/4 cup grated onions.
- 1 egg
- Two tablespoons of ketchup.
- One teaspoon of dried parsley.
- A half teaspoon of salt.
- 1/4 teaspoon black pepper.
- Two large sweet potatoes, peeled and diced
- Two teaspoons of coconut oil.
- 1/4 cup unsweetened almond milk.
- 1/4 teaspoon nutmeg.
- 4 cups of trimmed green beans.
- Garnish with additional ketchup, fresh parsley, etc.

Instructions

- Preheat the oven to 180°C (160°C fan-forced) and lightly butter a 9x5-inch loaf pan.

- In a large bowl, combine turkey, breadcrumbs, onion, egg, ketchup, parsley, salt, and pepper. Transfer the mixture to the prepared loaf pan and form into a loaf.
- Bake for 40 minutes, or until the meatloaf is fully cooked and reaches an internal temperature of 165°F.
- Cook the sweet potatoes in a large pot of boiling water until tender, about 20 minutes. Drain and return to the pot. Add the coconut oil, almond milk, nutmeg, salt, and pepper, and mash until smooth.
- Cook the green beans in a medium pot of boiling water for about 10 minutes, or until they are crisp tender. Drain and add salt and pepper to taste.
- Serve the meatloaf alongside the sweet potato mash and green beans. If preferred, garnish with more ketchup and fresh parsley.
- Pair your turkey meatloaf with sweet potato mash and green beans.

Nutritional values per serving:
- Calories: 400.
- Protein: 28 grams
- Vitamin A (260% DV)

Lentil Pasta Primavera with Parmesan Cheese

- **Servings: four.**
- **Prep time is 25 minutes.**

Ingredients

- 8 ounces of lentil pasta (penne or fusilli)
- Salt to taste.
- Two teaspoons of olive oil.
- 2 garlic cloves, minced
- Chop 2 cups of mixed vegetables, like broccoli, zucchini, and cherry tomatoes.
- One-quarter cup vegetable broth
- Two teaspoons of lemon juice.
- 1/4 teaspoon red pepper flakes.
- 1/4 cup grated parmesan cheese.
- Optional garnishes include fresh basil, more cheese, and so forth.

Instructions

- Cook the pasta in a large pot of boiling salted water until al dente, as directed on the package. Drain and return to the pot.
- Heat the olive oil in a large skillet over medium-high heat, then sauté the garlic for about 1 minute or until fragrant.
- Cook the mixed vegetables, broth, lemon juice, red pepper flakes, salt, and pepper, stirring periodically, until soft, about 15 minutes.

- Add the Parmesan cheese and stir to mix.
- Pour the pasta primavera over the lentil pasta and top with fresh basil and additional cheese, if preferred.
- Top your lentil spaghetti primavera with Parmesan cheese.

Nutritional values per serving:

- Total calories: 360.
- Protein: 18 grams
- Fibre: 12 grams.

Vegetarian Chili with Cornbread

- **Servings: six.**
- **Prep time is 50 minutes.**

Ingredients

- One tablespoon of coconut oil.
- 1 onion, chopped
- One red bell pepper, chopped
- 2 garlic cloves, minced
- Two teaspoons of chili powder.
- One teaspoon of cumin.
- 1/2 teaspoons of smoked paprika.
- Salt and pepper to taste.
- 1 can (28 ounces) of diced tomatoes
- One (15-ounce) can of black beans, drained and rinsed
- One (15-ounce) can of kidney beans, drained and rinsed

- One cup of veggie broth.

- Two tablespoons of tomato paste.

- One tablespoon of apple cider vinegar.

- Optional garnishes include shredded cheese, sour cream, and green onions.

- One (8.5-ounce) package of gluten-free cornbread mix.

- 1 egg

- One-third cup coconut oil

- 2/3 cup unsweetened almond milk.

Instructions

- Preheat the oven to 180°C (160°C fan-forced) and lightly butter an 8x8-inch baking pan.

- Heat the coconut oil in a large saucepan over medium-high heat. Sauté the onion, bell pepper, garlic, chili powder, cumin, smoked paprika, salt, and pepper until tender and fragrant, about 15 minutes.

- Add the tomatoes, black beans, kidney beans, broth, tomato paste, and vinegar, and bring to a boil. Reduce the heat and let the chili to simmer, uncovered, for about 20 minutes, or until thick and flavourful.

- In a large mixing bowl, combine the cornbread mix, egg, coconut oil, and almond milk until thoroughly blended.

- Place the mixture in the prepared baking sheet and bake for 20 minutes, or until brown and a toothpick inserted in the centre comes out clean.
- Serve the chili with cornbread. Garnish with cheese, sour cream, and green onions as desired.
- Pair your vegetarian chili with cornbread.

Nutritional values per serving:

- Calories: 560
- Protein: 16 grams
- Fibre: 14 grams.

Turmeric Tofu Stir-Fry with Brown Rice.

- **Servings: four.**
- **Prepare time: 30 minutes.**

Ingredients

- One block (14 ounces) of firm tofu, drained and pressed
- Two teaspoons of corn-starch.
- One teaspoon of turmeric.
- A half teaspoon of salt.
- 1/4 teaspoon black pepper.
- Two teaspoons of coconut oil.
- 2 tablespoons of minced ginger.
- 2 garlic cloves, minced
- 2 cups broccoli florets.

- One red bell pepper, sliced
- 1/4 cup coconut aminos.
- Two teaspoons of rice vinegar.
- One spoonful of honey.
- One tablespoon of sesame seeds.
- Optional garnishes include sliced green onions and minced cilantro.
- Four cups cooked brown rice.

Instructions

- Cut the tofu into bite-sized pieces and toss with corn-starch, turmeric, salt, and pepper until evenly coated.
- Heat the coconut oil in a large skillet over medium-high heat. Cook the tofu pieces, stirring regularly, until brown and crisp, about 15 minutes. Place the tofu on a platter and keep heated.
- In the same skillet, heat the ginger, garlic, broccoli, bell pepper, coconut aminos, vinegar, and honey until the mixture boils.
- Reduce the heat to a simmer, stirring periodically, for about 10 minutes, or until the veggies are crisp tender.
- Return the tofu to the skillet and toss to mix. Sprinkle with sesame seeds and, if preferred, add green onions and cilantro.
- Enjoy your turmeric tofu stir-fry with brown rice!

Nutritional values per serving:

- Calories: 480.

- Protein: 18 grams

- Calcium: 25% DV.

Salmon with Roasted Sweet Potatoes and Black Bean Salsa.

- **Servings: four.**

- **Prep time is 40 minutes.**

Ingredients

- Four (4-ounce) salmon fillets.

- Two teaspoons of olive oil.

- Salt and pepper to taste.

- Two teaspoons of dried oregano.

- Two large sweet potatoes, peeled and diced

- One (15-ounce) can of black beans, drained and rinsed

- 1/4 cup chopped fresh cilantro.

- Two teaspoons of lime juice.

- One-quarter teaspoon of cumin

- One-quarter teaspoon of garlic powder

- Optional toppings include avocado, feta cheese, pumpkin seeds, and more.

Instructions

- Preheat the oven to 200°C (180°C fan-forced) and prepare a baking sheet with parchment paper.

- In a small bowl, combine 1 tablespoon olive oil, salt, pepper, and oregano.

- Brush the salmon fillets with the oil mixture and arrange them on one end of the prepared baking sheet. Bake for 15 minutes, or until the salmon is well cooked and readily flaked with a fork.

- Toss the sweet potato in a large basin with the remaining 1 tablespoon olive oil, salt, and pepper until evenly coated.

- Spread the sweet potatoes evenly on the other end of the prepared baking sheet and bake for 20 minutes, flipping halfway through, until soft and golden.

- In a medium bowl, combine the black beans, cilantro, lime juice, cumin, garlic powder, salt, and pepper.

- Top the salmon fillets with the roasted sweet potato and black bean salsa. Add your favourite toppings and enjoy your salmon with roasted sweet potato and black bean salsa.

Nutritional values per serving:

- Calories: 440

- Protein: 30 grams.

- Fibre: 10 grams.

Chicken and Vegetable Soup with Whole Wheat Noodles.

- **Servings: six.**
- **Prep time is 40 minutes.**

Ingredients

- Two teaspoons of coconut oil.
- 1 onion, chopped
- Two carrots, peeled and sliced
- Two celery stalks, diced
- 4 garlic cloves, minced
- Salt and pepper to taste.
- Six cups of chicken broth.
- 2 cups shredded cooked chicken.
- 2 cups of mixed veggies, including green beans, corn, and peas.
- 2 teaspoons of freshly chopped parsley.
- 4 ounces of whole wheat noodles, like egg noodles or spaghetti.
- Optional garnishes include shredded cheese, sour cream, and other ingredients.

Instructions

- Heat the coconut oil in a big pot over medium-high heat. Sauté the onion, carrots, celery, and garlic for around 15 minutes. Season with salt and pepper to taste.
- Bring the broth, chicken, and mixed vegetables to a boil.
- Reduce the heat to a simmer, uncovered, for about 15 minutes, or until the vegetables are soft.
- Stir in the parsley and adjust seasoning as needed.
- Cook the noodles in a separate pot of boiling salted water until al dente, as directed on the package. Drain and add to soup.
- Garnish the soup with your preferred toppings and enjoy your chicken and vegetable soup with whole wheat noodles!

Nutritional values per serving:
- Calories: 320.
- Protein: 24 grams
- Fibre: 6 grams.

Shrimp Scampi with Zucchini Noodles and Cherry Tomatoes.

- **Servings: four.**
- **Prep time is 25 minutes.**

Ingredients

- Four medium zucchini spiralized or sliced into thin strips.
- Salt to taste.
- Two teaspoons of olive oil.
- One pound of big shrimp, peeled and deveined
- Two teaspoons of minced garlic.
- 1/4 teaspoon red pepper flakes.
- A quarter cup of white wine or chicken broth
- Two teaspoons of lemon juice.
- Two tablespoons of butter.
- 1/4 cup chopped fresh parsley.
- One cup cherry tomato, halved
- Optional garnishes include grated Parmesan cheese, lemon wedges, and so forth.

Instructions

- Place the zucchini noodles in a colander and season with salt. Allow them to drain for 15 minutes before squeezing off the excess water with paper towels.

- Heat the olive oil in a large skillet over medium-high heat. Cook the shrimp, garlic, red pepper flakes, salt, and pepper for about 10 minutes, or until pink and curled. Place the shrimp on a platter and keep heated.

- In the same skillet, combine the wine or broth and lemon juice and heat to a boil. Reduce the heat to a simmer, stirring occasionally, for about 5 minutes, or until slightly reduced.

- Stir in the butter and parsley, and season with extra salt and pepper as desired.

- Toss in the zucchini noodles and cherry tomatoes until combined. Cook for about 5 minutes, or until the noodles are well heated and the tomatoes are mushy.

- Serve the shrimp scampi over the zucchini noodles and cherry tomatoes, topped with cheese and lemon wedges if desired.

- Pair your shrimp scampi with zucchini noodles and cherry tomatoes.

Nutritional values per serving:

- Calories: 320.
- Protein: 28 grams
- Vitamin C: 50% DV.

CHAPTER 6

Snacks

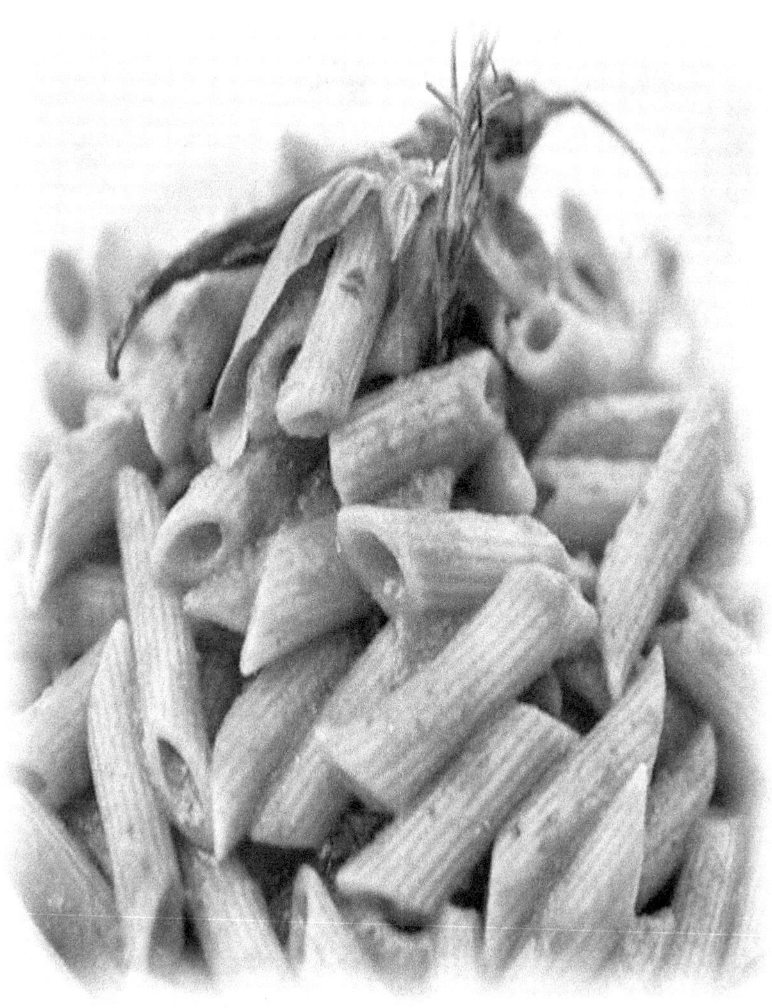

Vegetable sticks with Hummus

- **Servings: four.**
- **Prep time is 10 minutes.**

Ingredients

- Four cups of mixed vegetable sticks, including carrots, celery, cucumber, and bell pepper.
- 1 cup hummus (store-bought or homemade)

Instructions

- Wash the vegetables, chop them into sticks, and place them on a dish.
- Dip your vegetable sticks in hummus!

Nutritional values per serving:

- Calories: 160.
- Protein: 6 grams.
- Fibre: 6 grams.

Apple Slices with Almond Butter

- **Servings: two.**
- **Prepare time: 5 minutes.**

Ingredients

- One large apple, cored and sliced
- Two tablespoons of almond butter.

Instructions

- Wash, slice, and arrange the apples on a platter.
- Spread almond butter on apple slices and enjoy!

Nutritional values per serving:

- Calories: 200.
- Protein: 5 grams.
- Healthy fats: 12 grams

Fruit and Nut Mix

- **Servings: four.**
- **Prepare time: 5 minutes.**

Ingredients

- One-quarter cup raw almonds
- 1/4 cup raw walnuts.
- 1/4 cup dried cranberries.
- 1/4 cup dried apricots, chopped

Instructions

- In a small bowl, combine the almonds, walnuts, cranberries, and apricots.
- Store in an airtight container or divide into four servings and enjoy your fruit and nut mixture!

Nutritional values per serving:

- Calories: 220.
- Protein: 6 grams.

- Iron (10% DV)

Greek Yogurt with Berries and Chia Seeds.

- **Servings: two.**
- **Prepare time: 5 minutes.**

Ingredients

- One cup plain Greek yogurt.
- Two teaspoons of honey.
- 1/2 cup of mixed berries, including blueberries, raspberries, and strawberries.
- Two teaspoons of chia seeds.

Instructions

- In a small bowl, combine the yogurt and honey and whisk until smooth and creamy.
- Wash and chop the berries before adding them to the yogurt mixture.
- Sprinkle with chia seeds, then enjoy your Greek yogurt with berries and chia seeds!

Nutritional values per serving:

- Calories: 220.
- Protein: 14 grams.
- Calcium: 15% DV.

Hard-Boiled Eggs.

- **Servings: four.**
- **Prepare time: 15 minutes.**

Ingredients

- Four big eggs.
- Salt and pepper to taste.
- Optional toppings include mayonnaise, mustard, and paprika.

Instructions

- Gently lower the eggs into a medium pot of boiling water and cook for 10 minutes, or until hard cooked.
- Drain and rinse the eggs with cold water to stop the cooking process.
- Peel and slice the eggs, seasoning with salt and pepper to taste.
- Serve with your preferred toppings and enjoy your hard-boiled eggs!

Nutritional values per serving:

- Calories: 80.
- Protein: 6 grams.
- Choline: 25% of the daily value.

Rice Cakes with Avocado and Tomato.

- **Servings: two.**
- **Prep time is 10 minutes.**

Ingredients

- 4 rice cakes (plain or barely salted)
- One ripe avocado, peeled and mashed
- Salt and pepper to taste.
- One-quarter teaspoon of garlic powder
- One-quarter teaspoon dried basil
- 1/4 cup cherry tomatoes, halved
- Optional garnishes: lemon juice, fresh basil, etc.

Instructions

- In a small mixing bowl, mash the avocado with a fork and season with salt, pepper, garlic powder, and basil.
- Spread the avocado mixture on the rice cakes, then top with cherry tomatoes.
- Optional garnishes include lemon juice and fresh basil.
- Enjoy your rice cakes with avocado and tomato!

Nutritional values per serving:

- Calories: 240
- Protein: 5 grams.
- Healthy fats: 15 grams

Edamame pods.

- **Servings: four.**
- **Prep time is 10 minutes.**

Ingredients

- Two cups of frozen edamame pods.
- Salt to taste.

Instructions

- Cook the edamame pods in a medium pot of boiling salted water for 5 minutes, or until soft.
- Drain and season with additional salt to taste.
- Enjoy the edamame pods!

Nutritional values per serving:

- Calories: 120.
- Protein: 10 grams.
- Fibre: 5 grams.

Carrot Sticks and Guacamole

- **Servings: four.**
- **Prepare time: 15 minutes.**

Ingredients

- 4 large carrots peeled and sliced into sticks.
- Two ripe avocados, peeled and pitted.
- 1/4 cup chopped fresh cilantro.

- Two teaspoons of lime juice.

- Salt and pepper to taste.

- One-quarter teaspoon of cumin

- One-quarter teaspoon of garlic powder

- Optional toppings include diced onion, tomato, jalapeño, etc.

Instructions

- Wash the carrots, chop them into sticks, and place them on a dish.

- In a small mixing basin, mash the avocados with a fork. Stir in the cilantro, lime juice, salt, pepper, cumin, and garlic powder.

- Add your favourite toppings and stir thoroughly.

- Serve with carrot sticks as a dip and enjoy with guacamole!

Nutritional values per serving:

- Calories: 200.

- Protein: 4 grams.

- Vitamin A (210% DV)

Trail Mix with Dark Chocolate

- **Servings: four.**

- **Prepare time: 5 minutes.**

Ingredients

- One-quarter cup raw almonds

- 1/4 cup raw cashews.

- 1/4 cup dried cranberries.
- One-quarter cup dark chocolate chips

Instructions

- In a small bowl, combine the almonds, cashews, cranberries, and chocolate chips.
- Store in an airtight container or split into four portions and serve with dark chocolate!

Nutritional values per serving:

- Calories: 260
- Protein: 6 grams.
- Antioxidants: 4 grams

Homemade Energy Bites

- **Serves: 16**
- **Prepare time: 15 minutes.**

Ingredients

- One cup gluten-free oats.
- A half-cup of almond butter
- One-quarter cup honey
- 1/4 cup shredded coconut.
- Two teaspoons of chia seeds.
- One-quarter teaspoon of vanilla extract
- One-quarter teaspoon of salt

- Optional toppings: chocolate chips, dried fruits, almonds, etc.

Instructions

- In a large mixing bowl, combine the oats, almond butter, honey, coconut, chia seeds, vanilla, salt, and any additional ingredients.
- Chill the mixture for 15 minutes to firm up.
- Form the mixture into 16 balls and place in an airtight container in the fridge or freezer.
- Enjoy your homemade energy nibbles.

Nutritional values per serving:

- Calories: 120.
- Protein: 3 grams.
- Fibre: 3 grams.

CHAPTER 7

Desserts

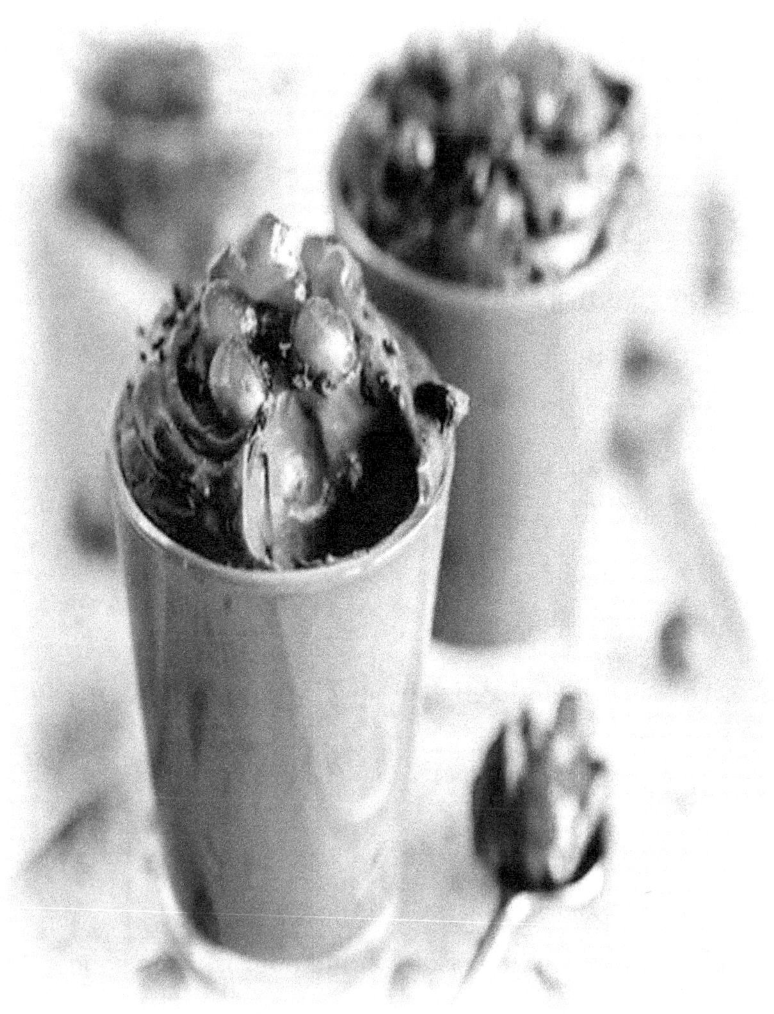

Fruit Crisp with Gluten-Free Crumble Topping

- **Serves: 8**
- **Prepare time: 45 minutes.**

Ingredients

- 4 cups of chopped fresh or frozen fruit, such apples, pears, berries, and peaches.
- Two teaspoons of honey.
- Two teaspoons of corn-starch.
- One teaspoon of vanilla extract.
- One-fourth teaspoon cinnamon
- One-quarter teaspoon of salt
- One cup gluten-free oats.
- One-quarter cup almond flour
- 1/4 cup chopped nuts (almonds, walnuts, or pecans)
- 1/4 cup melted coconut oil.
- Two tablespoons maple syrup.
- Optional toppings include whipped cream, ice cream, and yogurt.

Instructions

- Preheat the oven to 180°C (160°C fan-forced) and lightly butter an 8x8-inch baking dish.
- In a large mixing basin, combine the fruit, honey, corn-starch, vanilla, cinnamon, and salt until well combined.

Transfer the fruit mixture to the prepared baking dish and spread evenly.

- In a small bowl, mix together the oats, almond flour, almonds, coconut oil, and maple syrup. Sprinkle the oat mixture over the fruit mixture and gently press to adhere.
- Bake for 25 minutes, or until the fruit bubbles and the topping turns golden and crunchy.
- Top the fruit crisp with your favourite toppings and enjoy it with gluten-free crumble topping!

Nutritional values per serving:

- Calories: 260
- Protein: 4 grams.
- Fibre: 5 grams.

Dark Chocolate Avocado Mousse.

- **Servings: four.**
- **Prepare time: 15 minutes.**

Ingredients

- Two ripe avocados, peeled and pitted.
- 1/4 cup unsweetened cocoa powder.
- One-quarter cup honey
- 1/4 cup unsweetened almond milk.
- One teaspoon of vanilla extract.
- One-quarter teaspoon of salt

- Optional toppings include whipped cream, berries, and nuts.

Instructions

- In a food processor or blender, add the avocados, cocoa powder, honey, almond milk, vanilla extract, and salt.
- Process until smooth and creamy, scraping down the sides as needed.
- Transfer the mousse to a bowl and chill for at least an hour until thickened.
- Top the mousse with your favourite toppings and enjoy your dark chocolate avocado mousse!

Nutritional values per serving:

- Calories: 280.
- Protein: 4 grams.
- Healthy fats (18 g)

Baked Apples with Cinnamon and Nuts.

- **Servings: four.**
- **Prepare time: 45 minutes.**

Ingredients

- 4 big apples, cored and sliced
- Two teaspoons of honey.
- Two teaspoons of cinnamon.
- 1/4 teaspoon nutmeg.
- 1/4 cup chopped nuts (walnuts, pecans, or almonds)

- Optional toppings include whipped cream, ice cream, and yogurt.

Instructions

- Preheat the oven to 180°C (160°C fan-forced) and gently butter a 9x13-inch baking pan.
- In a large mixing bowl, combine the apple slices, honey, cinnamon, and nutmeg until well covered.
- Transfer the apple mixture to the prepared baking dish and spread it evenly.
- Sprinkle the nuts over the apple mixture, then bake for 20 minutes, or until the apples are soft and caramelized.
- Top the baked apples with your favourite toppings and enjoy them with cinnamon and almonds!

Nutritional values per serving:

- Calories: 200.
- Protein: 3 grams.
- Vitamin C: 15% DV.

Chia Pudding with Berries and Coconut Milk.

- **Servings: four.**
- **Prep time is 10 minutes (including overnight chilling).**

Ingredients

- 1/4 cup chia seeds.
- Two cups unsweetened coconut milk.

- Two teaspoons of honey.

- One-quarter teaspoon of vanilla extract

- One-quarter teaspoon of salt

- 1 cup of mixed berries, including blueberries, raspberries, and strawberries.

- Optional toppings include shredded coconut, almonds, and more.

Instructions

- In a medium bowl, combine the chia seeds, coconut milk, honey, vanilla, and salt.

- Cover the bowl and refrigerate overnight, or until the chia seeds absorb the liquid and form a pudding-like consistency.

- Wash and cut the berries and mix them into the chia pudding.

- Top with your favourite toppings and enjoy your chia pudding with berries and coconut milk!

Nutritional values per serving:

- Calories: 240

- Protein: 4 grams.

- Fibre: 10 grams.

Frozen Yogurt Bark with Berries and Nuts

- **Serves: 8**
- **Preparation time is 10 minutes (plus freezing time).**

Ingredients

- Two cups plain Greek yogurt.
- Two teaspoons of honey.
- One-quarter teaspoon of vanilla extract
- One-quarter teaspoon of salt
- 1/2 cup of mixed berries, including blueberries, raspberries, and strawberries.
- 1/4 cup chopped nuts (almonds, walnuts, or pistachios)

Instructions

- Line a baking sheet with parchment paper and set it aside.
- In a small bowl, combine the yogurt, honey, vanilla, and salt. Whisk until smooth and creamy.
- Spread the yogurt mixture thinly on the prepared baking sheet.
- Sprinkle the berries and nuts over the yogurt mixture and gently press to adhere.
- Freeze for a minimum of 4 hours, or until firm.
- Break the frozen yogurt bark into pieces and serve it with berries and nuts!

Nutritional values per serving:

- Calories: 120.
- Protein: 6 grams.
- Calcium (10% DV)

Homemade Fruit Popsicles

- **Serves: 8**
- **Prep time is 15 minutes (plus freezing time).**

Ingredients

- 2 cups of mixed fruit, such as mango, pineapple, and kiwi, chopped
- One-quarter cup water
- Two teaspoons of honey.
- One-quarter teaspoon of lime juice
- Eight popsicle melds and sticks

Instructions

- In a blender, combine the fruit, water, honey, and lime juice until smooth and frothy.
- Pour the fruit mixture into the popsicle molds, then insert the sticks.
- Freeze for a minimum of 6 hours, or until solid.
- Savour your homemade fruit popsicles!

Nutritional values per serving:

- Calories: 60.

- Protein: 1 gram.

- Vitamin C: 40% of the Daily Value

Dark Chocolate-Covered Dates

- **Serves: 16**

- **Prep time is 20 minutes (plus chilling time).**

Ingredients

- Sixteen pitted dates.

- One-quarter cup almond butter

- 4 ounces dark chocolate, chopped

- One teaspoon of coconut oil.

- Optional toppings include sea salt, shredded coconut, and chopped almonds.

Instructions

- Cut a slit in each date and fill with 1 teaspoon almond butter. Close the dates and lay them on a baking sheet covered with parchment aper.

- In a microwave-safe bowl, melt the chocolate and coconut oil in 30-second intervals, stirring between each, until smooth and shiny.

- Dip each date in melted chocolate before returning to the baking sheet.
- Sprinkle with your favourite toppings and chill for around 15 minutes to let the chocolate to solidify.
- Enjoy your dark chocolate-covered dates!

Nutritional values per serving:
- Calories: 120.
- Protein: 2 grams.
- Antioxidants: 2 grams

Baked Sweet Potatoes with Coconut Flakes and Spices.

- **Servings: four.**
- **Prepare time: 45 minutes.**

Ingredients
- Scrub four medium sweet potatoes and puncture them with a fork
- Two teaspoons of heated coconut oil.
- Two teaspoons of honey.
- One-fourth teaspoon cinnamon
- 1/4 teaspoon nutmeg.
- One-quarter teaspoon of salt
- 1/4 cup unsweetened coconut flakes.

Instructions

- Preheat the oven to 200°C (180°C fan-forced) and prepare a baking sheet with parchment paper.
- Arrange the sweet potatoes on the prepared baking sheet and bake for 40 minutes, or until soft and tender.
- In a small mixing bowl, blend the coconut oil, honey, cinnamon, nutmeg, and salt until thoroughly incorporated.
- Cut open the sweet potatoes and sprinkle with the coconut oil mixture. Sprinkle with coconut flakes and serve your roasted sweet potato with seasonings!

Nutritional values per serving:

- Calories: 240
- Protein: 2 grams.
- Vitamin A (260% DV)

Rice Cakes with Cinnamon and Nut Butter.

- **Servings: two.**
- **Prepare time: 5 minutes.**

Ingredients

- 4 rice cakes (plain or barely salted)
- 2 tablespoons of nut butter like almond, peanut, or cashew.
- One-fourth teaspoon cinnamon
- Optional toppings include sliced bananas, honey, and so forth.

Instructions

- Spread the nut butter on the rice cakes and sprinkle with cinnamon.
- Add your favourite toppings and eat your rice cakes with cinnamon and nut butter!

Nutritional values per serving:

- Calories:180
- Protein: 5 grams.
- Healthy fats: 9 grams

Fruit and Herbal Smoothie

- **Servings: two.**
- **Prep time is 10 minutes.**

Ingredients

- One cup plain Greek yogurt.
- A quarter cup of fresh mint leaves
- Two teaspoons of honey.
- One-quarter teaspoon of vanilla extract
- One-quarter teaspoon of salt
- 2 cups of mixed fruit, such as pineapple, mango, and kiwi, chopped
- 1 cup ice cubes.

Instructions

- In a blender, combine the yogurt, mint, honey, vanilla, and salt. Process until smooth and frothy.
- Blend the fruit and ice cubes until smooth and thick.
- Enjoy your fruit and herb smoothie!

Nutritional values per serving:

- Calories: 220.
- Protein: 12 grams.
- Calcium: 15% DV.

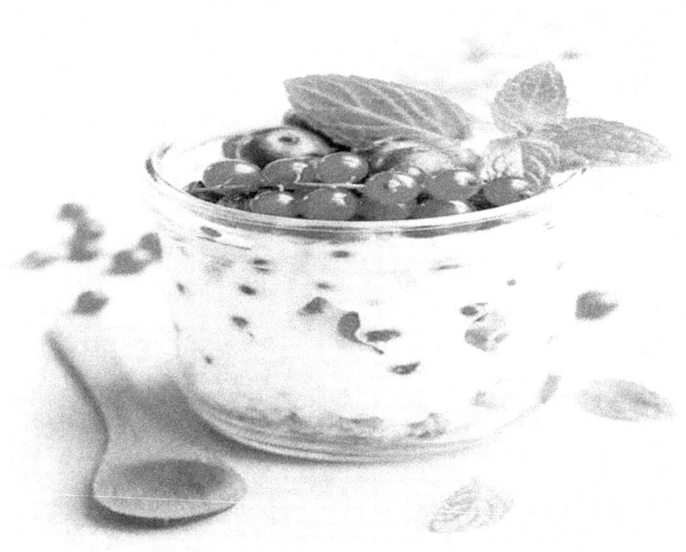

CHAPTER 8

Bonus

Tips for Cooking with Hashimoto's Disease

• **Select anti-inflammatory foods**. Inflammation is a major element in Hashimoto's disease because it destroys the thyroid and causes the immune system to attack it.

Fruits, vegetables, nuts, seeds, fish, olive oil, and herbs are all good sources of anti-inflammatory nutrients. Gluten, dairy, soy, sugar, processed meals, and vegetable oils can all contribute to inflammation. Aim to consume more of the former and less of the latter.

• **Avoid goitrogens**. Goitrogens are chemicals that can disrupt thyroid function by inhibiting the uptake of iodine, a mineral required for thyroid hormone production.

Cruciferous vegetables (including broccoli, cabbage, kale, and cauliflower), soy, peanuts, and millet are examples of common goitrogens. You do not have to fully avoid these meals, but you should limit them and prepare them thoroughly, as heat might deactivate some of the goitrogens.

• **Increase your selenium intake**. Selenium is another mineral that contributes to thyroid function by converting the dormant thyroid hormone T4 into the active hormone T3.

Selenium has anti-inflammatory and antioxidant qualities that can help protect the thyroid from harm. Foods high in selenium include Brazil nuts, sunflower seeds, eggs, mushrooms, and shellfish. Aim for approximately 200 mcg of selenium per day, which is similar to about two Brazil nuts.

• **Spice up your meals**. Spices may enhance the flavour of your dishes while also providing health advantages. They contain phytochemicals that can affect the immune system, reduce inflammation, and support thyroid function.

Turmeric, ginger, garlic, cinnamon, and rosemary are among the most effective spices for Hashimoto's disease. You can use them to flavour meats, soups, salads, and desserts.

• **Create your own sauces and dressings**. Store-bought sauces and dressings may contain hidden sources of gluten, dairy, soy, sugar, and chemicals, which can cause inflammation and increase Hashimoto's symptoms.

Making your own sauces and dressings is simple and gives you control over the ingredients and flavour. To make your own dressing, combine olive oil, vinegar, lemon juice, honey, mustard, herbs, and spices. To make your own sauces, combine coconut milk, tomato paste, nut butter, and broth.

• **Try gluten-free grains and flours.** Gluten is a protein present in wheat, barley, and rye that can trigger inflammation and autoimmune in some persons with Hashimoto's disease.

If you are gluten intolerant, you should avoid it and instead use gluten-free grains and flours. Examples include rice, quinoa, oats, buckwheat, millet, amaranth, and tiff. To make your own breads, muffins, pancakes, and cookies, try almond flour, coconut flour, cassava flour, and tapioca flour.

• **Snack intelligently**. Snacking can help you maintain a stable blood sugar and avoid cravings and overeating. However, you should choose nutritious and delicious snacks over those heavy in sugar, salt, and fat.

Healthy snacks for Hashimoto's include fresh or dried fruits, nuts, seeds, hummus, guacamole, hard-boiled eggs, yogurt, and dark chocolate. You may also make your own energy bars, granola, and popcorn with gluten-free oats, nuts, seeds, honey, and spices.

Here are some suggestions and strategies for cooking with Hashimoto's disease. By following these guidelines, you can eat delicious and healthful meals that will benefit your thyroid and general health.

Four-Week Meal Plan

Week 1

Monday

- Breakfast: Antioxidant Smoothie Bowl
- Lunch is salmon salad with quinoa and roasted vegetables.
- Dinner is baked salmon with roasted Brussels sprouts and quinoa.
- Snack: vegetable sticks with hummus.
- Desserts: fruit crisp with gluten-free crumble topping.

Tuesday

- Breakfast: Scrambled eggs with avocado and smoked salmon.
- Lunch: Lentil Soup and Whole Wheat Bread.
- Dinner: Chicken curry with coconut milk and vegetables.
- Snacks: Apple slices and almond butter.
- Dessert: Dark Chocolate Avocado Mousse.

Wednesday

- Breakfast: Chia pudding with coconut milk and mango.
- Lunch: Chicken lettuce wraps with avocado and mango salsa.
- Dinner: One-Pan Lemon Herb Shrimp and Roasted Asparagus
- Snack: Fruit and Nut Mix.
- Dessert: Baked apples with cinnamon and nuts.

Thursday.

- Breakfast: oatmeal with berries and nuts.
- Lunch: Black bean burgers with gluten-free buns
- Dinner: Turkey meatloaf with sweet potato mash and green beans.
- Snack: Greek yogurt with berries and chia seeds.
- Dessert: Chia pudding with berries and coconut milk.

Friday

- Breakfast: Sweet potato hash with eggs.
- Lunch: Turkey and vegetable stir-fry with brown rice.
- Dinner: lentil pasta primavera with parmesan cheese.
- Snack: Hard-boiled eggs.
- Dessert: Frozen Yogurt Bark with Berries and Nuts

Saturday

- Breakfast: Quinoa porridge with cinnamon and apples.
- Lunch: Chickpea Salad Sandwich with Whole Wheat Bread
- Dinner: Vegetarian chili with cornbread.
- Snacks: Rice cakes with avocado and tomato.
- Dessert: homemade fruit popsicles.

Sunday

- Breakfast: Gluten-free pancakes with banana and nut butter.
- Lunch: Tuna salad with mixed greens and avocado.
- Dinner: Turmeric tofu stir-fry with brown rice
- Snack: Edamame pods.
- Dessert: Dark Chocolate Covered Dates.

Week 2

Monday

- Breakfast: Green smoothie with kale, apple, and ginger.
- Lunch: Quinoa salad with roasted sweet potatoes and black beans.
- Dinner: Salmon with roasted sweet potatoes and black bean salsa.
- Snack: Carrot sticks and guacamole.
- Dessert: Baked sweet potato with coconut flakes and spices.

Tuesday

- Breakfast: Baked tofu scramble with vegetables.
- Lunch: Leftover turkey and vegetable soup with whole grain crackers.
- Dinner: Chicken and vegetable soup with whole wheat noodles.
- Snack: Trail Mix with Dark Chocolate.
- Dessert: Rice Cakes with Cinnamon and Nut Butter.

Wednesday

- Breakfast: Coconut yogurt parfait with granola and berries.
- Lunch: Shrimp Scampi with Zucchini Noodles, Cherry Tomatoes
- Dinner: Baked apple with cinnamon and nuts.
- Snack: Homemade Energy Bites.
- Dessert: Fruit and Herb Smoothie.

Thursday

- Breakfast: Antioxidant Smoothie Bowl
- Lunch is salmon salad with quinoa and roasted vegetables.
- Dinner is baked salmon with roasted Brussels sprouts and quinoa.
- Snack: vegetable sticks with hummus.
- Desserts: fruit crisp with gluten-free crumble topping.

Friday

- Breakfast: Scrambled eggs with avocado and smoked salmon.
- Lunch: Lentil Soup and Whole Wheat Bread.
- Dinner: Chicken curry with coconut milk and vegetables.
- Snacks: Apple slices and almond butter.
- Dessert: Dark Chocolate Avocado Mousse.

Saturday

- Breakfast: Chia pudding with coconut milk and mango.
- Lunch: Chicken lettuce wraps with avocado and mango salsa.
- Dinner: One-Pan Lemon Herb Shrimp and Roasted Asparagus
- Snack: Fruit and Nut Mix.
- Dessert: Baked apples with cinnamon and nuts.

Sunday

- Breakfast: oatmeal with berries and nuts.
- Lunch: Black bean burgers with gluten-free buns
- Dinner: Turkey meatloaf with sweet potato mash and green beans.
- Snack: Greek yogurt with berries and chia seeds.
- Dessert: Chia pudding with berries and coconut milk.

Week 3

Monday

- Breakfast: Sweet potato hash with eggs.
- Lunch: Turkey and vegetable stir-fry with brown rice.
- Dinner: lentil pasta primavera with parmesan cheese.
- Snack: Hard-boiled eggs.
- Dessert: Frozen Yogurt Bark with Berries and Nuts

Tuesday

- Breakfast: Quinoa porridge with cinnamon and apples.
- Lunch: Chickpea Salad Sandwich with Whole Wheat Bread
- Dinner: Vegetarian chili with cornbread.
- Snacks: Rice cakes with avocado and tomato.
- Dessert: homemade fruit popsicles.

Wednesday

- Breakfast: Gluten-free pancakes with banana and nut butter.
- Lunch: Tuna salad with mixed greens and avocado.
- Dinner: Turmeric tofu stir-fry with brown rice
- Snack: Edamame pods.
- Dessert: Dark Chocolate Covered Dates.

Thursday

- Breakfast: Green smoothie with kale, apple, and ginger.
- Lunch: Quinoa salad with roasted sweet potatoes and black beans.
- Dinner: Salmon with roasted sweet potatoes and black bean salsa.
- Snack: Carrot sticks and guacamole.
- Dessert: Baked sweet potato with coconut flakes and spices.

Friday

- Breakfast: Baked tofu scramble with vegetables.
- Lunch: Leftover turkey and vegetable soup with whole grain crackers.

- Dinner: Chicken and vegetable soup with whole wheat noodles.
- Snack: Trail Mix with Dark Chocolate.
- Dessert: Rice Cakes with Cinnamon and Nut Butter.

Saturday

- Breakfast: Coconut yogurt parfait with granola and berries.
- Lunch: Shrimp Scampi with Zucchini Noodles, Cherry Tomatoes
- Dinner: Baked apple with cinnamon and nuts.
- Snack: Homemade Energy Bites.
- Dessert: Fruit and Herb Smoothie.

Sunday

- Breakfast: Antioxidant Smoothie Bowl
- Lunch is salmon salad with quinoa and roasted vegetables.
- Dinner is baked salmon with roasted Brussels sprouts and quinoa.
- Snack: vegetable sticks with hummus.
- Desserts: fruit crisp with gluten-free crumble topping.

Week 4

Monday

- Breakfast: Green smoothie with kale, apple, and ginger.
- Lunch: Quinoa salad with roasted sweet potatoes and black beans.
- Dinner: Salmon with roasted sweet potatoes and black bean salsa.
- Snack: Carrot sticks and guacamole.
- Dessert: Baked sweet potato with coconut flakes and spices.

Tuesday

- Breakfast: Baked tofu scramble with vegetables.
- Lunch: Leftover turkey and vegetable soup with whole grain crackers.
- Dinner: Chicken and vegetable soup with whole wheat noodles.
- Snack: Trail Mix with Dark Chocolate.
- Dessert: Rice Cakes with Cinnamon and Nut Butter.

Wednesday

- Breakfast: Coconut yogurt parfait with granola and berries.
- Lunch: Shrimp Scampi with Zucchini Noodles, Cherry Tomatoes
- Dinner: Baked apple with cinnamon and nuts.
- Snack: Homemade Energy Bites.

- Dessert: Fruit and Herb Smoothie.

Thursday

- Breakfast: Antioxidant Smoothie Bowl
- Lunch is salmon salad with quinoa and roasted vegetables.
- Dinner is baked salmon with roasted Brussels sprouts and quinoa.
- Snack: vegetable sticks with hummus.
- Desserts: fruit crisp with gluten-free crumble topping.

Friday

- Breakfast: Scrambled eggs with avocado and smoked salmon.
- Lunch: Lentil Soup and Whole Wheat Bread.
- Dinner: Chicken curry with coconut milk and vegetables.
- Snacks: Apple slices and almond butter.
- Dessert: Dark Chocolate Avocado Mousse.

Saturday

- Breakfast: Chia pudding with coconut milk and mango.
- Lunch: Chicken lettuce wraps with avocado and mango salsa.
- Dinner: One-Pan Lemon Herb Shrimp and Roasted Asparagus
- Snack: Fruit and Nut Mix.
- Dessert: Baked apples with cinnamon and nuts.

Sunday

- Breakfast: oatmeal with berries and nuts.
- Lunch: Black bean burgers with gluten-free buns
- Dinner: Turkey meatloaf with sweet potato mash and green beans.
- Snack: Greek yogurt with berries and chia seeds.
- Dessert: Chia pudding with berries and coconut milk.

CONCLUSION

As we complete this cookbook, I'm grateful for the opportunity to be a part of your Hashimoto's journey. Remember that persistence in embracing the Hashimoto's diet lifestyle is the key to long-term well-being. In addition to the ideas offered here, consult with healthcare specialists for tailored counsel.

Your input is valuable; it can encourage others. Please share your positive experiences. Thank you for letting me be a part of your healing path. I wish you good health and unlimited joy.

With Appreciation,

Christiana White.